T0257044

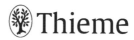

How NOT to Review a Medical Paper

A Very Short Manual

Markus K. Heinemann, MD, PhD
Editor-in-Chief
The Thoracic and Cardiovascular Surgeon
German Society for Thoracic and Cardiovascular Surgery
Cardiac, Thoracic and Vascular Surgery
Universitätsmedizin Mainz
Mainz, Germany

Thieme
Delhi • Stuttgart • New York • Rio de Janeiro

Publishing Director: Ritu Sharma
Director, Editorial Services: Rachna Sinha
Project Manager: Nidhi Chopra
Vice President Sales and Marketing: Arun Kumar Majji
Managing Director & CEO: Ajit Kohli

Thieme Medical and Scientific Publishers Private Limited.
A - 12, Second Floor, Sector - 2, Noida - 201 301,
Uttar Pradesh, India, +911204556600
Email: customerservice@thieme.in
www.thieme.in

Cover design: Thieme Publishing Group
Page make-up by RECTO Graphics, India

Printed in India by EIH Limited – Unit Printing Press

5 4 3 2 1

ISBN 978-93-88257-64-0
eISBN 978-93-88257-65-7

Important note: Medicine is an ever-changing science undergoing continual development. Research and clinical experience are continually expanding our knowledge, in particular our knowledge of proper treatment and drug therapy. Insofar as this book mentions any dosage or application, readers may rest assured that the authors, editors, and publishers have made every effort to ensure that such references are in accordance with **the state of knowledge at the time of production of the book**.

Nevertheless, this does not involve, imply, or express any guarantee or responsibility on the part of the publishers in respect to any dosage instructions and forms of applications stated in the book. **Every user is requested to examine carefully** the manufacturers' leaflets accompanying each drug and to check, if necessary in consultation with a physician or specialist, whether the dosage schedules mentioned therein or the contraindications stated by the manufacturers differ from the statements made in the present book. Such examination is particularly important with drugs that are either rarely used or have been newly released on the market. Every dosage schedule or every form of application used is entirely at the user's own risk and responsibility. The authors and publishers request every user to report to the publishers any discrepancies or inaccuracies noticed. If errors in this work are found after publication, errata will be posted at www.thieme.com on the product description page.

Some of the product names, patents, and registered designs referred to in this book are in fact registered trademarks or proprietary names even though specific reference to this fact is not always made in the text. Therefore, the appearance of a name without designation as proprietary is not to be construed as a representation by the publisher that it is in the public domain.

Again, this book must be dedicated to my scrutinizing teachers in editing as well as in writing a medical paper:

Hans Georg Borst,

who was always my first and most painstaking reviewer,

and

Hank Edmunds,

Former Editor of *The Annals of Thoracic Surgery*, who guided me through my early efforts as a reviewer for his journal with admirable patience.

Contents

溫故而知新，可以為師矣。
Reviewing what you have learned
and learning anew,
you are fit to be a teacher.

孔夫子 *Kong Fu Zi* - 論語 *Lunyu, ch. II*

1

Introduction

So you've finally made it. The Editor-in-Chief has invited you to become a Reviewer for the renowned *Journal of Asphaltology*. The welcome gift is a manuscript ambitiously titled "Risk factors to develop systemic asphaltosis: a multivariate analysis." You vaguely remember your case report "Pulmonary shadow revealed: a rare case of bronchial asphaltosis," an early effort which was accepted by that very journal 8 years ago after several revisions and considerable shortening. Now what?

Over the years, having written several papers and having read the relevant literature, you may have become rather experienced in how to write a medical paper.[1] But suddenly switching sides and looking critically at a manuscript written by somebody else seems like a totally different cup of tea. Luckily, the last author of the manuscript in question is your former teacher in asphaltology at Spandau University. So it can't be all bad. Or can it?

Speaking of asphalt: there are no such things as research into "serum asphalt" or "asphaltosis" and the like. The term was actually coined spontaneously by my teacher Hans Borst as a typical example for a useless and superfluous measure and has stuck in my brain ever since because of its absurdity. I regarded it perfect for the anonymization purposes it serves here.

This book intends to share tips and tricks about how to review a manuscript. Like its sister volume[1] it shows several negative examples in order to make you avoid the same pitfalls and mistakes. Positive experience is also illustrated. The most important prerequisite for a reviewer, however, is fairness. You must be willing to read and correct the pages in front of you from a neutral distance. Otherwise you are doomed to fail and will do the authors a disservice.

Declining an invitation to review is no disgrace. On the contrary, there are numerous good reasons to do so. You don't have the time right now. You feel awkward about the subject. You feel biased (see Chapter 2). You just don't feel like it at the moment because there is trouble at home and you do not want to explain it. All of these are perfectly acceptable. For the Editor it is very helpful if you give him a brief idea. He can then proceed with the selection process and do you better justice the next time.

By the way, one (obligatory) remark regarding political gender correctness: the admittedly male author of this book has used the masculine form throughout the text. This by no means implies that female colleagues are considered unequal or even inferior. The primary aim for an author, however, must remain readability. The much requested gender-neutral phrasing severely impairs exactly that. Sorry.

2

Forms of Peer Review

Peer review is an established way for journals to have a submitted manuscript evaluated by experts familiar with the field of research. Editors usually recruit their reviewers from their author pool, applying selection criteria such as experience and authorship of especially "good" manuscripts, although definition of the latter may be a subjective judgment. Furthermore, colleagues familiar from essential networking are added. For papers of a more interdisciplinary nature, it is helpful to know specialists beyond one's own field. Recently, specialized search tools for editors have become available through the electronic manuscript processing systems (publons.com/benefits/reviewer-connect).

😲 Bad Example

Manuscript title: "High resolution PET scanning for detection of atypical asphaltomas—a novel C14-tracing technique"

Selected reviewers:

1. Martin Blackpool, MD, MSc, Professor of Asphaltology, Lancashire University Hospital, Preston, UK

2. Prof. Dr. Alfons Tegtmayer, Professor für Asphaltologie, Rhein-Herne-Universität, Castrop-Rauxel, Germany

Problem:

Two clinical asphaltologists, no expert from radiology or nuclear medicine involved.

There is a continuing debate in the publishing world how best to avoid bias during peer review, mostly concerned with "who should know what?".

The most common form used by the majority of journals is called "single-blinded peer review."

2.1 Single-Blinded Peer Review

In this type of review, the invited reviewers do know the authors and institutions where the manuscript comes from. Their comments, however, are sent back blinded to the authors, granting (only) the reviewers' anonymity. This modality may abet self-interest. If the reviewer senses competition in his own field of research, a suggestion to reject or to at least revise substantially may clear the field. Personal animosities can also be fought under cover. If an Editor is well informed, as he should be, he will not invite potential adversaries. On the other hand, asking dependent individuals may only provoke inappropriate adulation.

😞 Bad Example

Manuscript title: "Carboliximab as a new treatment modality in disseminated asphaltoma." Senior author: Martin Blackpool,

MD, MSc, Professor of Asphaltology, Lancashire University Hospital, Preston, UK

Invited reviewer (knows authors): Prof. Dr. Alfons Tegtmayer, Professor für Asphaltologie, Rhein-Herne-Universität, Castrop-Rauxel, Germany

Recommendation: "By all means accept. This promises to become a seminal work in the future treatment of asphaltomas."

Problem:

Alfons received all his training in asphaltology from Martin and owes him his current position.

2.2 Double-Blinded Peer Review

In double-blinded peer review, the reviewer is also blinded to the origin of the manuscript. In theory this seems fairer to the authors and should facilitate a more neutral reviewing process. Strict anonymity of the manuscript is mandatory, which often means a cumbersome process to be done by the Editorial Office before the manuscript can be sent out. Not many journals are willing to follow that path, although there is evidence that the quality of the reviews is effectively higher.

😜 Good Example?

Manuscript title: "Carboliximab as a new treatment modality in disseminated asphaltoma." Senior author: Martin Blackpool, MD, MSc, Professor of Asphaltology, Lancashire University Hospital, Preston, UK

Invited reviewer (blinded to authors): Prof. Dr. Alfons Tegtmayer, Professor für Asphaltologie, Rhein-Herne-Universität, Castrop-Rauxel, Germany

Recommendation: "Reject. The authors are obviously not overly familiar with the specific intricacies of the treatment strategies for this rare disease."

Problem (?):

Martin is also the author of the standard textbook "Fundamentals of Asphaltology." Alfons received all his training in asphaltology from him. Apparently the manuscript is well below standard because Alfons did not even suspect its origin.

2.3 Open Peer Review

Open peer review is the other extreme in which all names are known to everybody. This is used by more revolutionary editors who propose that this modality will encourage an even more open discussion. Some do publish the reviewers' remarks along with the paper. As this is still regarded as unconventional by the majority of those involved, it will take a while before its advantages can be judged. The beginning looks promising.[2]

2.4 Preprints

As an extreme of the extreme, so-called "preprint servers" have already become an accepted publishing modality in the basic sciences. Here manuscripts are openly accessible to everybody for comment before they have gone through peer review. This is supposed to foster scientific discussion, allowing the paper to mature during the whole process. For clinical medicine, preprints remain highly controversial for various reasons.[3]

The modality of the peer review process is determined by the Editor-in-Chief of the respective journal—who by nature has to know everything. That makes him the one in charge. It is his obligation, however, to guarantee maximum neutrality to all involved. For this person, in turn, absolute independence of employers, societies, industry, or publishers is mandatory. Easier said than achieved (see Chapter 10).

3

Basic Principles: What to Look for (...in the Different Parts of a Manuscript)

Basically, you should approach reviewing a manuscript much as you would start simply reading it. Usually the invitation to review will already have provided you with the abstract, in this case making you accept to do so. If the abstract is written well it has raised certain expectations because you should have the basic information regarding the content. It is best to go through the paper step by step, although starting with a curious look at the Conclusions is probably just as well.

Occasionally you may realize that you have seen this particular abstract/paper before, it having been submitted to a different journal for which you also review. This normally means that it has been rejected there, hopefully following your recommendation. In this case you should notify the Editor. More often than not you will still be asked to review it, and to check if the text has been modified in any way, for instance according to your suggestions, or if it has been resubmitted unchanged. This is vital information for an eventual decision (see also Chapter 8).

For you personally, this situation is actually quite flattering because it shows that you are really considered a true expert by different editors. But remember: it's a small world after all.

When you have had a good glance at the manuscript and feel that you are capable of reviewing it, it is very helpful for authors, editors, and yourself to analyze it step-by-step.[4] If you feel unsure or even have a conflict of interest, you must decline to review and also give the Editor the reason why you did so.[5]

3.1 Abstract

This is the part you already know and which made you inquisitive for more. So it should be concise and interesting and contain the most important data. It is highly recommended, however, to compare the numbers given in the Results section to those given in the Abstract. Sometimes they do not match. If the absolute numbers in the text are markedly higher, it may well mean that you are reading an updated version of something that was rejected somewhere else before. More often, however, there are only small discrepancies. There should/must not be any! This always connotes very bad news for the authors because any inconsistency needs an explanation, at the same time raising concerns about scientific accuracy and integrity.

A decision to decline an invitation to review based on reading an Abstract implies either that you do not feel confident about your expertise, or simply that the Abstract alone is so poor that you do not want to see the rest. Letting the Editor know the reason will help him a lot.

3.2 Introduction

The Introduction is meant to lead the reader from the general to the specific: "Where do we come from, and where does this research (hopefully) lead us?" Please check if the authors have met this goal. Only the most relevant literature on the subject so far should be cited here. There is no need to tell a long story about the dim and distant past, but a brief statement about what we do know today is to be given instead, and why this led to further research, namely the presented one. A well-defined hypothesis is considered mandatory at this stage. The reviewer must check if there is one, and if so, if it is of relevance.

Ideally this is delineated in the last sentence of the Introduction: What was the purpose of the presented study, and what is it the authors wanted to investigate? Sometimes a brief glimpse whether the authors' expectations were eventually met or not is also given. It is an editorial decision if this is wanted here. The Editor will definitely welcome your opinion on that.

3.3 Methods

Although undoubtedly the most boring part to read, this is really the heart of the matter. The main question to be asked is: Was the study design adequate to test for the hypothesis? More often than not it was not, or only partially so.

In an experimental setting, the information given here must enable another researcher in a laboratory across the world to repeat the experiments and to get the same results. So the devil is in the details.

Clinical studies have the principal problem that they are conducted in a chaotic environment called daily life and are therefore prone to inaccuracies. In order to overcome or avoid these as much as possible, different study designs have been developed.

A typical hypothesis for a medical study is that one therapy is superior to another one. This is to be determined by a difference of a specific outcome measure, called the primary endpoint. A pretty good one is death, one might think, because there should be little debate over it. Far from it: there is a whole assortment of deaths in the medical literature, clad in important-sounding phrases: "early" or "late mortality," "in hospital" or "30 day mortality," "mid-term" or "long-term survival." "Survival" sounds much better but in fact also counts the dead. All endpoints must be clearly defined—and the definitions critically scrutinized by the reviewer.

😕 Bad Example

"This study investigated the long-term survival of patients receiving the new asphalt-covered Carboxa heart valve prosthesis (Group A) compared to the conventional, non-asphalt covered Shard model (Group B)... 2-year survival was 98/100 for Group A vs. 97/100 in Group B ($p = 0.999$)... Implantation of the Carboxa valve can be recommended because long-term survival is not inferior to the Shard valve."

Problem:

The Shard valve is known to last for 10 to 15 years on average. Thus, a definition of 2 years as "long-term" is completely useless if not fraudulent. The conclusion as given above is misleading to say the least.

The primary endpoint can be accompanied by several secondary ones meant to support the former. Again, the reviewer must check if these are selected appropriately with respect to the hypothesis, and if there are any confounding factors which may have influenced the result or its interpretation.

Even the most junior researcher has learnt that "prospective" studies are preferable to "retrospective" ones, but definitions may be hazy. A prospective study is one which has been designed before any of the study subjects (usually read: patients) had a chance to develop any of the outcome measures, that is, before the treatments were started. Anything else is retrospective. A classic teaser, very popular in surgery, is the pompous sounding "retrospective analysis of prospectively gathered data": "Let's have a look at our last 100 asphaltomata…" This is simply retrospective because the outcomes (dead, alive, crippled, whatever) had already happened when the study was initiated. That the data were collected "prospectively" is banal, because the parameters have simply been measured over time—and lifetime has a prospective direction only.

Real interventional clinical trials must be prospective by nature. An intervention (drug, device, operation, specific medical product) is applied to a subset of patients and the outcome compared to a (hopefully) comparable group which undergoes something else. The gold standard would be a randomized controlled trial (RCT) which has the highest impact in the realm of "evidence-based medicine," because only random assignment can guarantee an even distribution of known and unknown (!) characteristics between groups, thereby allowing conclusions about the causality of an intervention. Most journals demand that RCTs are done according to the CONSORT statement (www.consort-statement.org) and the necessary checklist and flowchart be submitted with the manuscript—for the reviewer (and Editor) to check. A clear declaration of the randomization method is very important. The famous "surgeon's preference" is certainly not a valid one. All RCTs should also be registered in national or international study registries.

Prospective cohort studies are much more popular because they are much less laborious. Their evidence level is lower and they are called "observational." Reviewers must be aware that "observational" is not meant as an automatically negative characterization. Especially in surgical specialties a true randomization is very hard to explain to potential participants, often making a statistically sensible recruitment in a reasonable time period impossible. It may be better to go for the next best thing, a prospective cohort study. The lack of a randomization increases the danger that known and unknown patient characteristics are unevenly distributed between the groups to be compared. In order to check for these unwanted effects, elaborate multiple regression analyses can be performed. "Propensity score matched groups" can adjust (only) for known potentially confounding factors and thus render groups more comparable. Again, the statistical effort must not be underestimated but at least the investigators can go ahead with their study and do the adjustment as they go along.

Another practical option is a "matched pair analysis" in case control studies. For this, each individual of a treatment group is assigned an otherwise similar "match" for comparison. For instance, if you treat a fair-haired 35-year-old woman of normal height and weight with your new intervention you need a similar person in the control group. This process, however, renders the data "dependent" rather than independent, which in turn limits their validity.

3.4 Statistics

A lot of the above already had to do with the correct application of statistical methods. Your average researcher in medicine will, however, have an MD degree, not one in mathematics. As medical school in most countries still follows a scientific curriculum, this should include a basic teaching in statistical models and principles. Reviewers and authors theoretically share these prerequisites. As long as you are still familiar with the basics of descriptive analysis of variance, Pearson's Chi-square, Fisher's exact, and the *t*-test, you should feel rather comfortable with a basic evaluation.

It is fairly easy to judge, for instance, if a measured variable is normally (or normatively) distributed and can therefore be given as a mean value +/− its standard error, or if it is not and therefore the median +/− the interquartile range should be given instead.

"The larger the better" is also a statistician's credo, because the magnitude of the all-important *p*-value, which signals a statistically significant difference or lack thereof, heavily depends on the sample size. One should have a feeling if a study is underpowered and, if in doubt, be able to check it. On the other hand, minimal differences may gain statistical (!) significance in huge sample sizes. The question remaining is: do these elaborate findings have any clinical relevance? Always remember that in medicine we are dealing with the lives of human beings and not with the attributes of elementary particles.

😃 Good (Impressive) Example

Accuracy of ASPHALT, CARBON, and NewWorldSCORE II scores was evaluated according to calibration and discrimination in terms of early postoperative mortality.

1. Calibration: Calibration can first be assessed by calculating the observed/expected mortality ratio (O/E ratio) obtained by dividing observed by expected mortality. An O/E ratio above 1 means underestimation of mortality and an O/E ratio below 1 means overestimation of mortality. In this series, the ratio was 1.79 for the ASPHALT score (overestimation), 0.63 for the CARBON score (underestimation), and 1.63 for NewWorldSCORE II (overestimation).

    The Hosmer–Lemeshow and the Spiegelhalter tests were also used to assess calibration. One has to keep in mind that the logistic regression model is simple, probably too simple, to account for many kinds of data. In this series, the authors report that predicted mortality based on the three models showed a positively skewed distribution. The qualitative interpretation of the skew is complicated. The skewness does not determine the relationship of mean and median. Possibility of several distributions may be evoked. I therefore believe that the p-values reported in the sentence "In these cases, the median rates of mortality predicted by ASPHALT, CARBON, and NewWorldSCORE II models were 1.8% ($p = 0.002$), 1.9% ($p = 0.003$), and 1.5% ($p = 0.0002$), respectively" are meaningless.

2. Discrimination: The concordance (c) statistics are the most commonly used performance measure. For a binary outcome, c-statistic is identical to the area under the receiver operating characteristic (ROC) curve. c-statistic of 0.5 denotes a zero ability to discriminate (the model is not better than chance at predicting the outcome). A c-statistic between 0.7 and 0.9 is a reasonable value and a c-statistic value over 0.9 denotes an excellent discriminative power. A c-statistic of 1 indicates a perfect discrimination. In this series, c-value is under 0.7 for ASPHALT and CARBON and attains 0.74 for NewWorldSCORE II.

One may therefore conclude that the accuracy (calibration + discrimination) of the three scores reported in this series is inadequate (insufficient).

Statistically, if this series is to constitute a reliable benchmark, the three models, inaccurate for this series, should undergo calibration to fit the studied population.

This is a (slightly abridged) original review by our faithful reviewer Nicodème Sinzobahamvya who is a pediatric cardiac surgeon, not a mathematician. He has his hobbies, as you can see, and he is NOT our biostatistical advisor. Here's another one for you, this time by Dietmar Boethig, who does have that position in our journal:

🫢 **Good (Impressive) Example**

"...Differences in score calibration or discrimination problems regarding certain types of asphaltoma treatment may be seen from 2 points of view (like a dog wagging its tail and vice versa):

1. The score can be 'blamed' for O/E differences ('poor calibration,' 'bad prediction' ...).

   Or:

2. The difference may simply be regarded as a difference between one's own results and the results in the score creator's often large (and thus representative) construction data set.

Both AsphaltScores indeed derive from a large multicenter data collection and coincide with results of many other asphaltology units. This view would indicate that the score-applying hospital has special strengths or weaknesses compared to the group of hospitals which contributed to the score construction. Since the hospital populations are usually much smaller than the score creator's construction data set, the latter point of view should be considered appropriate in the majority of cases—also in the presented manuscript."

Wow again! Please do not regard yourself underprivileged if you feel that you could never have written these reviews. Simply keep your threshold low for referring any judgment of statistical methods used in a study to a (professional) statistician. Most journals have them on hand and will have involved one anyhow, because the Editor felt overstrained and at a loss himself. Just stick to your medical background and judge the medical content—plus the clinical relevance, please.

3.5 Results

When the hopefully adequate methods have eventually produced results, these must be presented. Often there is wealth of data gathered. They may be best shown in tables and/or figures rather than in endless string sentences. If so, a repetition or duplication in the text must be avoided.

As a reviewer please judge if the tables are arranged in a logical way and that they are not too overbearing. A rule of thumb says that a table should fit on a regular journal page in a font size readable without a magnifying glass. If there is just too much information, it is advised to split one table into smaller ones.

In graphical depiction of results, one should be aware of under- or overscaling, meaning a distortion of the actual facts by adapting the scales of the respective axis. Line or field distinction should be distinctive, enabling reproduction in black/white/shades of gray. An appropriate use of color should also be remarked upon, especially if a journal still has to charge for color figures. In the case of pictures, a patient must not be identifiable and consent to use the picture(s) is mandatory, although this falls under the Editorial Office's obligations. Legends to all illustrations must be provided and should give all necessary information to understand what is being shown (only). They should not overflow into little paragraphs of their own.

The results section must present the findings in a neutral way. Anything judgmental is out of place, for instance phrases like "surprisingly," "as was to be expected," "logically," etc. Absolute numbers are a necessity to be supported by percentages if meaningful.

If a study shows that an assumed hypothesis is null and void, this is often declared as "failed research," and negative results tend to be unpopular with Editors. This is a mistake, because numerous examples show that an (unexpected) failure to prove something may actually be a valuable contribution to a totally different insight.[6] Always bear in mind that we do learn a lot from our errors, perhaps even more than from our successes. This is a bit like the philosophy behind this book. The mere fact that authors came up with a negative result is definitely not a reason to reject a paper. Publishing it will in fact probably prevent someone else to embark on the same futile journey again and ultimately conserve resources.

Definitely useless for a specialized journal are results which have been known and proven for a long time and will not contribute anything new to the informed reader. If the manuscript is otherwise sound and written well, the recommendation could be to submit it to a more general continuing education journal.

Good Examples (Two reviewers on the same manuscript)

Reviewer 1:

The authors present a single-center, retrospective observational report of 249 patients undergoing resection of an asphaltoma. Main findings are that tissue-sparing techniques are clinically superior to radical surgery, that the two patient populations differ in terms of baseline clinical parameters, and that the extension of the asphaltoma determines the surgical approach.

What is new about that? The content of the manuscript simply describes well-established truths about asphaltoma surgery.

Reviewer 2:

The authors report their experience and short-term outcomes on patients operated for asphaltoma.

For a retrospective analysis, 249 patients treated over 6.5 years is not a huge number.

Detailed pathologies and treatment modalities (except "tissue-sparing" and "radical" surgery) are not provided.

In summary, the manuscript tells us nothing new but only already known facts on asphaltoma resection, patient selection, choice of surgical modalities, etc.

Bad Example

The topic is of major interest since growing numbers of elderly people suffer from asphaltomata and the literature is silent about this topic.

However, the present study does not even fulfill the minimal criteria in methodology, hypothesis, and the presentation of the results.

Sorry but I cannot recommend the publication of this manuscript.

Problem:

That may all be very well, but it does in no way tell the authors how they might improve their manuscript.

3.6 Discussion

This is the part in which the findings have to be placed into context with the literature already known. Unfortunately it often gets mixed up with the Results section and vice versa. A good Discussion may start with a brief (!) summary of the findings and then lead to a comparison with what was published before. Here the authors can and must state if their study was contradictory or confirmatory and maybe even if this was anticipated or not. It is definitely very bad style to quote extensively from the referenced papers word-by-word. This is not plagiarism if done correctly, but simply very hard to read and unnecessary. A concise summary of the reference in question is more suitable. Moreover, this quoting should not be done in an endless lined-up fashion telling the reader about article after article after article, but should summarize and directly juxtapose their own results: same, different, why? It has to be evaluated if the most relevant references have actually been discussed or ignored (see also Chapter 3.8).

If not required in a separate section, potential limitations or shortcomings of the study also belong to the Discussion as well as possible alternative interpretations of the findings.

It is the reviewer's task to comment on the general logic and the coherence of the authors' interpretations. One's own opinion and experience may play a role here, but it is important to refrain from prejudice and be open to new insights. Reviewing a manuscript is a learning process for oneself.

3.7 Conclusions

The last part of the Discussion or a separate section will express the conclusions which in turn must give the basic information concerning the relevance of the study performed, and if its results will change the world or at least a little bit of it. It is amazing how many manuscripts remain uncertain or even ignorant about this most important part. The reviewer must double check if any conclusions made are indeed supported by the data given, or if they rather belong to the realm of unjustified speculation. An unwanted but frequent and unfortunate mistake is to conclude global uncertainties from some actual findings.

Good Examples (By three reviewers concerning the same manuscript)

Reviewer 1:

No causality is derivable regarding the development of asphaltoma or any other thoracic disease from these descriptive and incomplete and only moderately defined data as a correct control group is missing.

Reviewer 2:

In the introduction and discussion the focus of the manuscript seems lost at several occasions.

The authors then conclude that the incidence of asphaltoma depends on BMI and serum asphalt levels. However, there is no indication that the suggested causal relationship may be more than a speculation. The authors also conclude that further pulmonary effects seem to be associated to inflammatory processes. The reviewer was not able to identify any further pulmonary effect reported. Thus, the second part of the conclusion is also not supported by the results.

Reviewer 3:

Has the knowledge of the serum asphalt levels changed the clinical practice in the authors' institution and if so, how? The reviewer finds that hard to imagine.

It is obvious that not every study published will have a marked impact on the clinical practice of the future, but it should at least potentially be able to. Many manuscripts, however, such as the one severely criticized above, are nothing but a compilation of data fed into a statistics program and then presented more or less impressively to sell loose associations as scientific discoveries. For the reviewer such a ruse should be easily identifiable, although authors do become increasingly skillful in wrapping rubbish. This sad development must be blamed on the "publish or perish" mentality and the inappropriate attitude of many institutions to regard quantity as a quality measure.

3.8 References

As already mentioned in Chapter 3.6, the most relevant references must be cited and discussed. Although their selection may be subjective to a certain degree, there is usually a common consensus on which papers can be regarded seminal. Depending on the subject of the research, a time-span of about 5 to 10 years backwards is sufficient for a clinical manuscript.

In the basic sciences, 5 years ago is often regarded as having been in the Middle Ages and references have to be much more current. This has led to the creation of preprint servers with all their potential drawbacks for the sake of acuity (see also Chapter 2).

Reviewers must refrain from trying to place their own work under the cover of anonymity unless it really does fulfill criteria of relevance.

Bad Example (By A. Tegtmayer)

Can you please compare your technique also to a recently published article: Tegtmayer A et al. Asphaltoma resection employing the infrasound scalpel. J Asphaltol 2019; 64: 211–223.

4

A Matter of Style
(How to Say Nasty Things
in a Polite Way)

"It's called 'style', dear. You wouldn't understand."
(Basil Fawlty, addressing his wife Sybil, regarding an "object d'art" to be hung on the wall of the Fawlty Towers reception.)

😞 Bad Example

At a first glance there could be the aspect of an interesting presentation of a very important topic. But on a second glance it is not really at the level of a scientific publication.

Though 180 patients means a big number, we don't get information about the period, we don't get information about a randomization, we don't get information about decision criteria for operative/conservative treatment.

What about lateral thoracotomy (how many?)? What is a "severe asphaltoma"? How many patients have been dealt with surgically? You report about an unusually high number of complications in the conservative group. What exactly was your "conservative treatment"?

According to my experience over decades, this kind of asphaltoma presentation doesn't exist.

Could continue, but don't like to do so.

Even if the manuscript is totally below standard, it is the reviewer's duty to refrain from derogatory or even insulting remarks under the protection of presumed anonymity. The Editor still knows the identity and, again, has the duty to avert abusive reviews from the poor authors. This is usually done by finding someone else to review and by ditching the offender from one's database, ideally letting the person know why.

Bad Example

Would you be really knowledgeable about efficiently dealing with asphaltoma, you would not propose such a procedure.

Some manuscripts do indeed lack vital information and, depending on the journal's editorial management, many of those will be rejected without undergoing a review at all (see Chapter 6.5). But a few will always escape the Editor's critical eyes and enter the process. Rather than writing that it is all bad, it is much more helpful for the (obviously inexperienced) authors to get some advice how to improve their work. If it appears to be not salvageable, do let them know the reasons.

In case of a revision, it is perfectly alright for an author to state as follows: "Thank you for your comment, although we would have appreciated some more helpful criticism how to improve the quality of the manuscript." This takes some self-assurance, but if it is justified it should even help the apparently somewhat superficial reviewer to do better the next time—and not to feel hurt and suggest to reject the revision.

At the other end of the spectrum, when a reviewer really does like a manuscript, this should also be explained—probably even more to the Editor than to the authors. My favorite how-NOT-to positive review, however, is the following (definitely no joke!):

😕 Bad Example
Well done!

It may make the authors happy but is totally useless. Interestingly enough, in the above example the second reviewer recommended "major revision," listing several shortcomings to be amended.

The general approach to the wording of a review should be just like that for a scientific article, which it is in a certain way. Neutral phrasing and a descriptive rather than a judgmental attitude are to be employed. In official credentials it has become an unwritten rule to use nothing but positive wording. "The employee was always eager to meet the various demands." Everybody knows that this means "total failure." This hypocrisy stems from a concern to avoid litigation by all means. As this has not really to be feared in the review process of a journal, the language may and should be more honest including negativisms, but not insulting.

Good Example (As an alternative to the Bad Example presented earlier: "Would you be..." [p. 32])

It appears that the authors are still in the process of establishing an asphaltoma unit. Therefore publication of their results at this stage must be regarded as premature.

Good (Polite) Example

The reported results in general do not support further application of the described technique in this specific setting.

Meaning

You should stop doing this.

Although the major language to publish in has been English for quite some time now, people still do speak different languages as they may not be living in a primarily English-speaking country. Even the definition of the latter is a matter of debate, with some Etonians regarding the United States not to be one. Apart from such sophisticated discussions, the fact remains that most manuscripts are written by people for whom this is a second (or even third) language.

Bad Example
Terrible English. Hardly comprehensible.

Good Example
Although this reviewer is not a native speaker himself, he feels that the English language should be significantly improved.

More often than not the quality of the language is assessed independently by the Editorial Office before a manuscript enters the review process. If it is found to be of really inferior quality, a decision of "reject for language reasons" may be made, encouraging the authors to seek (professional) help. There are numerous means to get your thoughts translated into proper English. Unfortunately, almost all of them cost money, which in turn may be well spent.

Decision Based on Language Quality
I do realize that English is not your native language. As the manuscript in its present form contains numerous spelling and grammatical errors, it is very hard to follow your argument and the scientific content tends to get lost. I suggest that you have the text checked by a (near-) native speaker or a professional agency before resubmission of a corrected version, giving the ms-# of this one as a reference.

If the content of a manuscript is comprehensible and the majority of the flaws are of a grammatical nature, some publishers will still accept it and have the language "polished" during the copyediting process. Unfortunately, such a service has become rather uncommon due to increasing money restraints. By no means is it the duty of a reviewer to correct any language mistakes. A general, neutrally phrased remark suffices, and many journals have a separate "English" box to tick on their evaluation form. When remarks on language are made part of the general review, care should be taken to get them right to avoid embarrassment.

Bad Example (sic!)
The English words used are sometimes uncommonly.

Bad (Unnecessary) Example
I have some minor corrections to suggest:

page 5, line 34: "Patients who were unable (instead of inability) to give informed consent, had a (insert a space) known allergy…"

page 7, line 14: No wound infection (instead of infections) was observed.

Page 7, line 21: There are two full stops (..) at the end of the paragraph.

Finally a word on attitude. Whereas a reviewer can expect that authors have checked their manuscript for obvious typos, authors often get a review which looks like it has been hastily typed into a smartphone on a moving train. This is probably a realistic scenario and may be understandable given the lack of time we all experience.

One should, however, bear in mind that a sloppily written text will suggest a rather superficial perusal of the manuscript both to the authors and to the Editor. Please do give the review a "once-over" before clicking "submit."

😴 Bad Example

The authors evaluated the prognostic value of the high sensitivity serum aspahlt for the outcome after CARB scheme treatmnt. They found that the highsensitivity serum asphatl predicts the outcome (30 day mortality).

In General, this work represents a good step to further increase safety for the CABR scheme. There are, however some Points that Need to be adressed:

1. Please specify the in and exclusion criteria more precisly (concomittant operations allowed? etc.
2. The cummulative mortality exceeds the cumulative CARB score- is there an Explanation?
3. What is the bioavailability of asphalt? If the time between traetment and the Evaluation of serum asphatl the next day differs to much, this might have a great Impact in your results (2nd round the operationg day leads to a much shorter postoperative asphalt day 1). Did you perfomr any suplmentary blood samples? Maybe a time Frame of serum asphalt Levels after CARB would be interesting (intraoperativly, and every 4 hours?
4. Did you conclude any changes in Terms of managment if high Levels of serum aspahlt were detected? for example heparine? Aspirin ?

5. Any postoperative furhtr diagnostic experiences? Measuring the Levels of asphalt s one Thing, but drawing the right conlcuisons for complications of CARB is more essential. What are your criteria for a postoperative CT scann in Terms of ECG canges, asphalt, carbobodehydrogenas Levels? What would be the cut of for aspahlt Levels for a postoperative CT meaning a complication?

6. What is the influence of kkidney function o the asphatl Levels?

In General this work is a good step Forward in increasing saftey in CARB treetment however, we Need to draw the right conlusions...

Too much bonhomie and encouragement are also out of place.

🙁 Bad Example
Good luck with your paper, and thanks again for submitting it.

If the authors need luck for their manuscript it should probably be a "reject," and it would be the Editor's role to express gratitude for a submission.

5

How (Not) To Put It All Together

Now that you have read the manuscript and ideally written down some remarks, you are ready for the final step: wrapping it up nicely.

Most journals provide two different boxes for the entry of comments:

1. Confidential Comments to the Editor
2. Comments to the Authors

And those should be used accordingly. Please do *not* copy and paste a detailed review meant for the authors into the Editor's section—or, probably more important, vice versa. "Confidential" means that you can say things to the Editor you do not want to say to the authors, even under the protection of your anonymity, but still feel to be important.

Supposed wrongdoing may be such a reason. If you are not really sure whether the authors have copied from Tegtmayer's seminal work, you should at least mention the possibility to the Editor. If you have recognized your own work in the manuscript or can definitely prove plagiarism, this must, however, also be noted in the "Comments to the Authors" section to show them that they have been unmasked.

Good Example (Comments to the Authors)

This reviewer was very surprised to read his own words in the Discussion section (pg. 8, lines 14–26). The extensive section in question (12 lines!) is a word-by-word copy from my publication XY which is, in fact, given as a reference (# 8) somewhere else but not in conjunction here. I consider this a severe case of plagiarism and must base my recommendation to reject the manuscript on this finding alone.

The "honest opinion" is also meant for the confidential comments to the Editor. Even if you have done your best to be courteous and encouraging to the authors in their (in your opinion) total failure, you can be frank to the Editor to drive home the message you really wanted to give, most often "forget it!"

Good (Honest) Example (Comments to the Editor)

I have to stop reading (and writing my review) as I am finding mistakes over mistakes—it will make me burst if I do not.

As much as I love to read literature on serum asphalt levels and their role as a perioperative risk factor in our surgical area, the more I am shocked by manuscripts like this one.

The authors mix up several catchphrases without logical background. Biological correlations are completely misunderstood.

Their statistical analysis does not enable any conclusion. The small number of patients is the smallest problem, and it would not even be a problem if the authors would have given stringent data.

News value is extremely low if existent at all. Thus, I do not expect that this manuscript will ever be publishable.

An ideal review for the authors should be organized a bit like the scientific manuscript itself. Briefly summarize your opinion like in an Abstract, then go through the individual parts step-by-step, weighing their pros and cons, thus commenting on all major aspects of the design and methodology. Check the literature discussed for adequacy and judge if the conclusions drawn can really be based on the findings. And whether they are relevant.

A distinction between "major" and "minor" points is also helpful. The recommendation given to the Editor must NOT be part of the comments to the authors. From the text alone they should be able to guess the reviewer's opinion, and it is only the Editor's verdict which counts anyway (see Chapter 7).

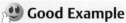 Good Example

Confidential Comments to Editor

Dear Editor,

- Please see below my detailed comment to the authors. Beyond this allow me to summarize my review in the following confidential remarks:
  - There is no obvious scientific or clinical relevance as this therapy for asphaltoma is already widely used.
  - The manuscript is overcrowded with duplicate or irrelevant information.
  - The language is rather catastrophic (many spelling errors, mutilated sentences, abundant use of abbreviations).
  - The two latter points render the text nearly unreadable.

I regret that, even with a benevolent attitude, I cannot recommend the manuscript for acceptance.

Comments to the Authors

Major

Between 2016 and 2018, the authors have identified 76 cases of asphaltoma (28 male, 48 female) out of a total of 1,360 patients with thoracic tumors. The patients were divided into two different treatment groups: group I = CARB regimen, $n = 40$; group II = conventional surgery, $n = 36$. There were no differences between groups regarding demographic data, operative data, or other basic characteristics. However, clinical outcome was much worse in group II in terms of hospital stay, patient satisfaction, thrombosis, and other short-term complications.

Unfortunately, there are several shortcomings. I shall elaborate on the most important of these in the following.

First, the data were taken from a time interval in which the CARB regimen should already have been the standard approach in asphaltoma treatment. This is valid for all manifestations. Furthermore, minimally invasive techniques were also widely introduced during this period and should likewise have helped to overcome the surgical problems seen in group II. In this respect, the general scientific relevance of the reported particular topic is rather low.

The language style and quality of the manuscript are largely insufficient. It does require extensive rewriting with correction of wording and sentence structure. Apart from this, the Results section is a nearly complete duplication of the data in the Tables. It is so overcrowded with information that it is almost unreadable.

There is a lot of reference to certain data not provided in the text or tables. For example I could not find the linear regression data (i.e., the risk factor analysis) referenced at the end of the Results section (page 8, lines 3 to 8). The numeric patient satisfaction scores are also not provided, neither in the Abstract (page 1, lines 26 to 27) nor in the text (page 8, lines 8 to 11). Besides, no further explanation of the scoring system is given. We also do not get any information about possible additional medical therapy and its efficiency.

On the other hand, some of the data are dispensable and do not contribute to the findings of the study. For example, the detailed description of the different anatomical variations of the lung segments is not relevant (page 9, line 37 to page 10, line 24).

The study was retrospective in nature. It still remains unclear how the patients were allocated to one of the treatment groups (i.e., CARB vs. conventional). Did the team apply well-defined criteria, or was the therapeutic strategy decided at random? Was this done identically in all three centers?

Minor

There are some more formal aspects:

- The Abstract provides no sufficient summary of the results (it only refers to hospital stay and patient satisfaction; the latter never appears in the manuscript).
- Definitions of asphaltoma stages should be given. Which classification is meant by stage III or IV?
- Fig. 3 is irrelevant.
- Fig. 6 might be dispensable, but this would be for the Editor to decide.
- The legend of Table 5 is incorrect ("Pain score pre and post operation"). The pain score does not appear in the manuscript.
- The legend of Table 6 is incorrect ("Hospital course data in both groups of patients"). This legend refers to Table 5 instead.

- Table 6 (the linear regression model) is referenced in the text (page 8, line 8) but not shown.
- Table 7 (satisfaction score) is referenced in the text (page 8, line 12) but not shown.
- There is inconsistent wording for the therapeutic modality in group I (CARB regimen, CARB scheme, "multimodality treatment").

With this detailed information the authors should be able to perform a thorough revision of their manuscript. For the Editor it is absolutely clear that this is not to be published and is most likely already a revised version of a manuscript previously submitted and rejected somewhere else. The inconsistencies in the table legends as well as the missing parts are typical indicators for that.

If needed, in many journals even regularly, manuscripts are sent to a statistical advisor to check the validity of the mathematical models used. Such reviews may then have their own style by nature, often requiring the Editor to read them more than once to fully comprehend them (see also Chapter 3 with examples). Again, the information given should be sufficient for the authors' statistician to improve that part.

Sometimes it is the reviewers, just like authors, who need a little nudge by the Editor who knows they can do better.

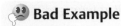 Bad Example

Comments to the Authors, First Version

The topic is of major interest since growing numbers of elderly people suffer from asphaltoma and the literature is rather silent about this topic.

However, the present study does not even fulfill the minimal criteria in methodology, hypothesis, and the presentation of the results.

Sorry, but I cannot recommend the publication of this manuscript.

Editor to Reviewer (After Rescinding the Review)

Thank you for your review. As reviews are supposed to help authors to do better the next time, especially in rejected manuscripts, it would be helpful if you could specify your critique. This can still be short but should be focused. Thank you for your cooperation and understanding.

Review (After Revision by the Reviewer)

The present work deals with a very important topic: the influence of tissue quality on possible asphaltoma development.

The authors correctly present the methods of tissue density measurement and analyze a monocentric collective of patients with asphaltoma. These were evaluated by CT for singular asphaltoma and multiple asphaltomata and the tissue density was determined in each case. Different analyses were carried out between different subgroups, each with a small number of patients.

Unfortunately, the manuscript lacks a scientific structure. There is no hypothesis, and no endpoints are defined.

Although the statistical tests may have been formally correct, the subgroup analysis cannot lead to the presented conclusion.

The authors show long-known facts with the presented results that older people have a weaker tissue and are hospitalized more often. However, it cannot be concluded from this analysis that multiple asphaltomata correlate with lower tissue density. The collective would have to be analyzed according to clearly defined subgroups and defined parameters, e.g., major/minor asphaltoma stage and age groups as well as tumor manifestation with age distribution, etc. In any case, a multifield table would have to result, which then has to be checked statistically. Here, however, the small number of cases will have a negative impact and a valid statement is unlikely to be allowed. Alternatively, a matched-pair analysis could be effective. I recommend to completely rework the study, involving a statistician.

Even if a detailed explanation is certainly helpful for the authors, it may well be that only a few words suffice to give a clear message to both editor and authors.

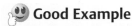 Good Example

Comments to the Editor

This is a nicely written report about extra-anatomic treatment for complex asphaltoma by a well-known group which has published about this subject before. This fact basically sums up my review: good series, nice pictures, nothing new. If you deem it original enough for the *International Asphaltology Journal,* fine—but again: it has all been said before.

Comments to the Authors

This is a nicely written case series reporting the group's experience with extra-anatomic treatment for complex asphaltoma manifestations. The techniques used are described in sufficient detail and illustrated well. Introduction and Discussion are somewhat on the rambling side.

The main critique, however, is that the group has basically said it all before. Even this fact notwithstanding, the whole article does not offer anything new for a specialized asphaltology journal. For a more general readership, it would be an excellent historical overview.

6

The Recommendation

A recommendation is a recommendation, not the final word. Decisions are made by Editors, hopefully based on recommendations. Therefore, the verdict by the reviewer should be stated in the space provided. Most journals offer the following options:

Accept / Minor Revision / Major Revision / Reject,

commonly with a respective box to tick. Apart from doing that, which is mandatory, one can use the confidential message to the Editor to drive home one's point.

😞 Bad Example (In Comments-to-the-Authors)
This article cannot be published in its present form.

😞 Bad Example (Complete Text of Comments-to-the-Authors)
Even though this is only a single-center retrospective study with a smaller number of patients, this is a nice hypothesis-generating observation.

The topic is important since beta-blocker therapy may hold the potential to significantly prolong asphalt degradation.

Therefore this study will for sure be of interest to the readers of the *Journal of Asphaltology*.

Recommendation (Ticked in box)

Minor revision

Editor and authors will ask the same question: "What should be the subject of the revision?" It is clear that this review including its recommendation is completely useless.

 Bad Example

Dear author, thank you for your submission which I have read with interest.

You report 92 patients (2004–2016) with an asphaltoma and the application of the CARB scheme therapy which were analyzed retrospectively. The patients were divided into an asphaltoma stage I group ($n = 72$, group A) and an asphaltoma stage >I group ($n = 20$, group B).

In group A, 15 patients had to be excluded because the CARB scheme was not employed. Additionally, group A was divided into three subgroups depending on the duration of treatment.

The conclusion was that a longer CARB treatment results in a longer hospitalization, regardless of the asphaltoma stage. Unfortunately, no explanation is given as to why different lengths of CARB treatment were needed for group I and its three subgroups, although all of them were classified as stage I.

Since group B consisted mainly of more advanced cases, the need for a prolonged CARB treatment is regarded self-explanatory.

There are numerous review articles in circulation that demonstrate that the duration of a CARB regimen of more than 14 days should be avoided, and that the therapy regimen should be reconsidered in cases apparently needing a prolonged application. In 2014 carbostyl-dinitrate was added to the CARB scheme. This constitutes a change in methodology. As such these patients must be excluded from the study, or at the very least form a separate group.

Due to deficits in the basic scientific procedure, I have to decline a publication of your article.

Although it is fairly apparent that there were serious flaws in the study design, the Reviewer is not in a position to decline a publication. The expression "basic scientific procedure" sounds impressive, presumably on purpose, and, in this context, pretty bad, but is completely unspecific—rendering everybody at a loss.

It may help a reviewer to learn about the definitions what the recommendations to the Editor (not to authors!) listed above actually mean.

6.1 Accept

This should only be used for manuscripts which can be published as they are. The need of insignificant language editing does not preclude it. In general, this option as a first decision is exceedingly rare, even for manuscripts invited by the Editor. In case of a revised manuscript (see Chapter 8) this signals that the reviewer is completely satisfied with the modifications made.

6.2 Minor Revision

The overall content and structure as well as the study design are all fine. Some additional information, however, may be helpful to understand the results or to comprehend the conclusions, or some rephrasing should be done. This option is also fairly common in cases of a Major Revision coming back with some points unattended to. The reviewer can put it at the Editor's discretion if a revised version should be sent back for a second review or if the final decision can be made in the Editorial Office based on the corrections done.

6.3 Major Revision

There is no fundamental flaw in the study design but more essential information is needed to judge the validity of the results and conclusions. Further statistical analysis or even additional data may be asked for. A remark similar to "The analysis should be recalculated excluding the patients with asphaltoma stage III as those constitute a completely separate entity" sounds more like being on the border of "Reject." Again, it is a recommendation. For the Editor it may be enough to put the thumb down, also depending on the other recommendation(s).

6.4 Reject

The study has simply too many shortcomings to allow publication and even a thorough revision is unlikely to save it. In the case of revised manuscripts, essential questions raised upon the former submission remain unanswered and an eventual satisfactory explanation remains highly unlikely. The ratio of all manuscripts rejected by all manuscripts submitted is the "rejection rate" of the journal which characterizes its selectiveness. In very sought-after, high-submission, and high-impact publications such as the *New England Journal of Medicine* or *Nature* it may be way above 90%. In the average clinical journal it is usually in the 60 to 70% range.

6.5 Rejected without Review

This is an Editorial Office decision made before a manuscript is even sent out for review, colloquially known as the "sudden death" option. An analysis of our own cases revealed five major causes of death in order of frequency:

> Invalid Category / Outside Scope of Journal / Lack of Originality / Faulty Science / Severe Language Problems

Whenever a reviewer complains about having been sent a pile of rubbish, a hopefully consoling answer is that the worst submissions which disqualify themselves at first glance have never gotten further than the Editor's desk. So who is the one to be pitied?

😊 Polite Recommendation

I thus feel the need to propose rejection of the submission.

Interestingly, the opinion of different reviewers and their subsequent recommendations tend to be rather unanimous. If this is the case, it makes the Editor confident to come to the right decision. A "major revision" and "rejection" combination, for instance, will usually lead to a rejection. With conflicting opinions an additional reviewer should be invited and the authors informed about a delay in the process. Many journals routinely look for an uneven number of referees, usually three, but for smaller, highly specialized ones it may be difficult enough to obtain two. It has been calculated that to get three opinions an Editor may have to send out up to eight invitations. This is, of course, the Editor's dilemma, but part of the job, as well as reading the important parts of each and every manuscript personally to form at least an impression if not an expert's opinion himself. The Editor's verdict will tip the balance in cases of doubt, so it must be well-founded on its own without having to be an in-depth review—another reason why ultrashort primary reviews are useless.

😊 Bad Example (Complete Review)

Nice study that hopefully represents a step to avoid asphalt implants in the future!

Recommendation

Accept

For the authors a decision of rejection is, of course, unpleasant. They will now have to decide if their study is definitely not worth publishing (rare) or if they should submit it somewhere else (frequent). If going the latter road, any helpful suggestion for improvement should be incorporated before resubmission, because any constructive criticism can only help. Moreover, especially in highly specialized fields, it may well be that the reviewer of the next journal has already reviewed it for the first one. If no changes have been performed according to the previous suggestions, this will inevitably lead to a quick and easy decision: another "reject."

Sometimes it is the Editor rather than the reviewer who becomes the target of frustrated authors. However emotional a reaction may be, it should always be taken seriously and answered.

😊 Good Example (Editor's Reply to a Complaint after Rejection)

Thank you for your enquiry. Your disappointment about a negative decision is understandable. In order to help you understand it better, let me answer your questions one-by-one:

"Our manuscript was left in your manuscript system for about 2 months and 10 days. We think that this period is very long for a journal."

This is correct for our journal but not for the majority of comparable scientific journals where even 3 months would be considered normal. The reason for the relative delay is explained below.

"We have noticed that our manuscript was reviewed by only one reviewer, although, in your system, you wrote that as a rule two referees are assigned to Original Articles."

The manuscript was sent for review to two reviewers on November 29. One did not respond adequately despite several reminders. In the end I based the decision on the one review which (as you know) was very critical but also very detailed and elaborate. This decision was also made in the interest of time so that it would enable you to send the manuscript somewhere else as early as possible.

"Could you tell me why this happened and could you tell me what one reviewer made with our manuscript for 2 months?"

I hope this is explained now. The reviewer who did the review was faster. The rest of time was lost trying to get the second one. Why reviewers do need time to review is a question which would have to be addressed to them.

"Also we thought that your reviewer was not blinded because he made a negative discrimination against us."

The reviewer was blinded as to where the manuscript did come from. This is our routine procedure. He did, in fact, point out shortcomings in detail in neutral phrasing and did not negatively discriminate you. I am not sure how you come to this assumption.

"We want to investigate these topics."

This you did.

"Also our manuscript has now to be reviewed by another reviewer(s)."

This is an editorial decision.

I hope that this explanation does shed some light on the fate of your manuscript. I advise you to follow the reviewer's comments regarding necessary revisions of your manuscript and submit it somewhere else, most logically to the *Journal of the Bavarian Society of Asphaltology* who gave you the grant.

7

If In Doubt, Shout!

Sometimes an invitation to review may cause uneasiness or at least raise questions. Is there a potential personal conflict of interest to review? Can one really consider oneself an expert on that topic? Isn't that a paper which bears an uncanny resemblance to one you just reviewed for somebody else? Or is it a rather boring sequel to the study which was published a year ago?

Another scenario is a manuscript which leaves the invited reviewer at a loss during reading. Be it that the text does not hold up to what title and/or abstract promised, be it that the methods employed seem questionable, or that (a rather common problem) the conclusions drawn somehow do not fit the results obtained. A third point of possible unease is at the recommendation stage, usually when a decision is to be made between major revision and rejection. Should one be forgiving or brutal?

In any case outlined above or any time you are in doubt how to proceed, just shout. To the Editor, that is. Most Editors know reviewers who call them almost on a regular basis because they want to discuss a specific aspect of a manuscript. This is something which should be supported and even encouraged. A brief oral discussion can make things so much easier. Email contact is, of course, also an option, maybe resulting in the Editor calling you.

Good Example

Reviewer's Enquiry

Honestly, I am not sure what to do with this paper. Is this a joke? The study design does not make sense. There is no structure, no proper methods or results, no figure legends. The conclusions drawn from the results do not make sense. It is very difficult and confusing to read.

Editor's Answer

Unfortunately it is no joke. The manuscript was on the verge of being rejected by me without review. On the other hand, infiltrating asphaltomata are a bit of a "hot topic" and I had the impression that the authors were really trying. If you feel that it is hopeless, just write so in your review. If we (most likely) reject it, it would still be helpful for the authors to learn what they have to do better next time, so it will be a learning process for them—another reason why I decided to send it out.

If a reviewer gets the feeling that he would really like to discuss a paper in public rather than just with the Editor, he may also suggest to write a commentary to be published along with the paper in case of acceptance. Sometimes this works the other way round: when an Editor reads a meticulous review he may ask the reviewer to complement the publication. Such additional comments are loved by readers, similar to the transcripts of oral discussions some journals add to the manuscripts backing a presentation at a congress. There is a feeling among editors that they may even increase the likelihood of a citation because the discussion is more comprehensive than usual.

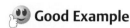 Good Example

Reviewer's Enquiry

I am chewing myself through the manuscript on VATS resection for asphaltoma. It is a good paper; everything it says seems true and relevant. The problem is not what they have written, but what they have left out. I do not believe that without turning the paper upside down and redoing all the statistics, they can add all data which may be necessary to give a complete picture of this controversial subject. What do you think of a commentary?

Editor's Answer

Thank you so much for taking care of that. Why don't you sum up your review so that they'll still be able to revise it? If it gets accepted in the end, we could then add an Invited Commentary by you. This should depict the whole scenario and will definitely enhance the visibility of the paper. Of course we must still wait what the other reviewers have to say. I'll keep you posted and look forward to your review.

8

Reviewing Revisions

😊 Good Example (Reply by Authors)

Enclosed, please find our revised manuscript titled, "Preoperative carbon-IV-score predicts post-operative atrial fibrillation after asphaltoma resection," for consideration in the *Journal of Asphaltology*. We appreciate the reviewer's thoughtful comments on our study. We believe the revised manuscript is stronger and more suitable for publication. In the manuscript, *we have addressed all of the points brought up by our reviewers*. In this letter, *we explain how we address the reviewers' concerns* and *additions we have made to our manuscript (in* red)... *(Followed by 12 point-by-point remarks and answers)*

😊 Good Example (Reply by Authors)

List of point-by-point responses to the referee comments.

Responses to Editor's Comments

We thank the Editor for this positive view of our work and the thoughtful and constructive comments. Corrections made in the text in response to these comments are highlighted in **red** color.

Responses to Reviewer #1

We thank the reviewer for this positive view of our work and the thoughtful and constructive comments. Corrections made in the text in response to these comments are highlighted in **green** color... *(Followed by an extensive list)*

😊 Good Example (Reply by Authors)

	Comment (Reviewer 1)	Answer
1	Clinically highly relevant study.	The authors would like to thank the reviewer for this comment.
2	Study population (page 4): "125 patients received asphaltoma resection plus LAA ligation..." but authors mentioned in introduction part that only group 1 (*n* = 57) received LAA ligation—clarification needed here; Exclusion criteria (page 5): concomitant surgery secondary to asphaltoma resection—which additional procedures? Minor aspect: would also recommend proof be read by native speaker.	We clarified the "study population" section in the revised manuscript as follows: "125 patients received asphaltoma resection either with or without LAA closure because of tumor and AF." We meant concomitant thoracic surgery procedures. The comment was considered in "exclusion criteria" section of the revised manuscript. The revised manuscript was edited by a native speaker.

	Comment (Reviewer 1)	**Answer**
3	Discussion (page 8): "ligation of LAA reduces ... stroke ... without additional procedural risks ..." Was this aspect studied in this population? Any differences noted in revision rate for bleeding, etc.? Needs clarification/ more precise wording.	We studied this aspect in this population but didn't clarify it well enough in the first version. There were no procedural risks regarding the LAA ligation such as bleeding. The comment was considered in the revised manuscript.

This is what you as a Reviewer (and Editor!) want. The authors have taken you seriously and are now giving you a point-by-point answer to your comments and questions. In case they could not provide required data they tell you why. In effect, all performed changes are commented and highlighted, any unchanged passages are explained. Sometimes this is even done in tabular form (see previous example). Unfortunately you do not get this too often, even if the journal's Instructions-for-Authors specifically ask for it. Apparently the interpretation of "point-by-point" can be a wide and diverse one.

😦 Nice Example (but Good?)

On the basis of your thoughtful, kind, and nice advice, I chose to rephrase the paper, and then resubmit to you. I believe this novel instrument has the potential to make a substantial contribution to asphaltoma surgery, either minimally invasive or traditional.

Thank you very much again for your caring help last time, and now I am expecting your further nice instruction.

If the answers given are satisfactory one may now suggest acceptance, if one feels completely ignored, rejection. It becomes more tricky when some parts have been perfected but others are still lacking, a situation frequently encountered, especially in cases where an extensive correction was required. This may then lead to the recommendation of a second revision, specifying again what still needs to be done.

Good Example

Comments to the Authors

Many thanks for revision and the answers. However, I still have one major concern: the incidence of observed events is very low. Based on the current data with less than 40 patients per group, no conclusion can really be drawn regarding safety. This limitation needs to be mentioned in the Abstract and Discussion sections. Again: no firm conclusion can be drawn based on the data, although their publication is strongly recommended by me. Your findings do add to the overall understanding of asphaltoma; it is your conclusions which simply cannot be drawn from them.

Editor, Then Requiring a Second Revision

The major problem with the paper is the low incident number—something which you cannot change. All conclusions must therefore be phrased very cautiously or deleted. Normally this does not suffice for a high-rank scientific publication. As your overall findings are definitely of interest for the asphaltology community, we would still publish it, but it must be stated very clearly that these are data merely in support of a theory, not a proof of it. The sentence that "further research is necessary" is normally disliked very much by editors. However, it needs to be included in this manuscript.

🙂 Good Example (Confidential Comments to the Editor)

In my opinion the authors provided an insufficient response to the concerns. The changes in the manuscript are only minor and my crucial questions have not been adequately answered in all cases.

If the authors additionally perform and evaluate a pre-operative CT scan, they should mention this in the text.

If they depart from the usual standard (i.e., the use of tangential clamping when performing the asphaltoma resection), they must further elaborate on this. They seem to always avoid tangential clamping and perform the procedure under full-thickness clamping, which increases tissue trauma.

Therefore, I suggest that the authors adapt their discussion accordingly before a possible publication (please see my detailed comments to the authors).

When reviewing such a revision of a manuscript one has seen before, a reviewer should definitely focus on the previously asked questions or comments. Any new ideas crossing the mind upon the second reading are only human but unfair to the authors. When asking for a second revision which raises completely new points, the Editor can expect to receive expressions of justified frustration or even chagrin by the authors.

😟 Bad Example (Extract from Authors' Reply, in Total More Than 2,000 Words in Length!)

...Unfortunately, the second review by the same reviewer lacks focus to some degree. I'm ready to do some changes proposed. But if he insists on each and every change he proposes then I must defend my viewpoint and say that I think that the reviewer did not completely understand the message of the manuscript. As an expert I can really understand how deep someone's understanding is, but I cannot automatically change my draft following each and every comment, particularly if I feel that the reviewer lacks focus at some points and now brings up something that is not really relevant or appropriate for this study and manuscript.

Dear Editor, please advise: I'm ready to do further changes in the manuscript to some parts but will not do all the changes and follow all the comments the reviewer gave, especially the new ones. When looking at the revised draft, the text has already been markedly changed, suggesting our compliance to the reviewer's previous comments. We can further alter some sentences but only to some degree. Noteworthy, the other reviewer seemed to be perfectly OK with the first version.

In conclusion, I think the reviewer stepped beyond the scope of a review, lacking the focus this time. Some comments given do address parts of manuscript which have already been changed as per the first suggestion, and I see no point to keep changing for changing's sake...

9

A Matter of Speed
(How Fast Is Too Slow?)

😃 Good Example

Dear Editor, first of all, thank you very much for the fast review process of your journal. This is a completely new experience for us, and we are looking forward to publishing our further work with you.

😞 Bad Example (Editor's Reply to an Enquiry)

Thank you for your enquiry. I am very sorry that this has happened again. I have reminded the reviewer pointing out the delay you had to experience with the original submission and do now hope that he will respond very soon.

Feedback like yours should enable me to amend our reviewing process in the future. Please accept my apologies that you have to suffer through this again.

The average reviewer is a busy doctor/scientist who commits himself to do reviews on top of the daily work. This is a voluntary service for which not much of a reward can be expected (see Chapter 10.5). It is therefore understandable if this task keeps moving down on the to-do list. Authors, on the other hand, are often also pressed for time because they need to see their paper published to gain academic credit, etc. Conflicts of interest between both parties are bound to happen. The Editor as the one in the middle has to do everybody justice.

There are few obligations more cumbersome than chasing reviewers because the submission system has sent another alert "review xx days overdue." On the other hand, scientists have come to expect a speedy service, although the definition of what constitutes "fast" may be vague. This is where the predatory journals come in, promising peer review and eventual publication within time-spans of 3 weeks or so. Everybody in the business knows that this is simply not possible for an ordinary manuscript in an ordinary journal with ordinary reviewers. Impatience may lead authors down a dangerous track and in order to prevent this, respectable journals should do their best to keep their workflows fluent and efficient. When asking authors about their expectations, a short time until the first decision is almost on top of the list.[7] Authors should, however, bear in mind that a really quick decision is likely to be negative. An efficient peer review process has become an important quality feature for journals.

From the Editor's angle, it is much easier to live with a "decline to review" signal than with an "accept-to-review" with no apparent consequence. The manuscript can then be assigned to somebody else, hopefully saving everybody's time. The automated submission systems send reminder e-mails to reviewers who are late, sometimes to no avail. The Editor still has to keep track and must finally intervene by assigning somebody else, which could have been done weeks earlier if the originally invited person had not been too open-hearted at the beginning. Repeated severe delays may also lead to exclusion from the reviewer pool, not exactly an elegant way out. Most submission systems offer an option for reviewers to define periods of unavailability, unfortunately an underused feature.

Another common boilerplate in an invitation-to-review e-mail is something like "If you are unable to review at this time, I would appreciate you recommending another expert reviewer." When used, this can be extremely helpful for the Editorial Office, potentially extending the pool of reviewers for good and thus helping to distribute the ever-increasing load on more shoulders.

"How fast is too slow, then?" you may ask. This, in turn, depends on the manuscript in question. First submissions will need a longer time than a quick check of changes in a minor revision. Original articles and elaborate analyses are more laborious than a short How-to-do-it or a Case Report. "Please try your best to complete your review within the next 2 weeks" is the average request, with the automatic reminders then setting in 3 weeks after the agreement to review.

A realistic time-span for a first-time submission of an original article is 3 to 4 weeks. Major revisions may be just as time-consuming as the original version, whereas it is hard to comprehend for an Editor why a short communication or a minor revision cannot be judged within 7 to 10 days. Again, if the invitation comes at an inconvenient time, a simple "decline" is probably the best solution. With extensive revisions this would, however, be really unfair. If authors have taken the trouble to incorporate the meticulous suggestions of a reviewer, there is almost an intrinsic moral obligation to re-review. Inviting a new reviewer at this stage is something Editors hate, because the new person will not be familiar with the manuscript and may have completely different views and ideas.

In general, journals which achieve an average of 1 month for a first decision are considered to be well managed.

😞 Bad Example

Enquiry to Editor

Dear editor: I delivered a clinical article titled "Asphaltoma resection combined with superior vena cava replacement" on August 3, 2017. Nearly 20 days have passed. I still find the status of the article as "under review." I hope you can tell me the current situation. I will be most grateful if you could let me know the current status of the manuscript. Please also advise if you need any additional information. Thank you very much for your consideration. I look forward to hearing from you soon.

Reply by Editor

Thank you for your enquiry. I am not sure if you are familiar with the process of serious peer review. It is not unusual for a well-founded review to take more than 3 weeks, especially during a time of the year when most of our reviewers are on holiday.

Should the timeframe not meet your expectations you are welcome to withdraw your manuscript.

Reply by Author

I felt very guilty when I received your letter. I will not choose to withdraw the manuscript. I will continue to wait patiently until the journal has reviewed my article. Please forgive my recklessness. Thank you again for your patience and reply.

10

The Journal and You

10.1 The Editor

The interface between the reviewer and the authors and the journal is the figure in the center, commonly known as the Editor (-in-Chief). He or she has the overall responsibility, both for the content and for the processes. The publisher and/or owner expects high quality, unfortunately often still measured by the Journal Impact Factor; authors want speedy and efficient handling of their efforts; reviewers are dependent on how many invitations they get and for which articles. Everybody should expect a maximum of integrity.

Not surprisingly, the Editor is usually a somewhat senior person with a long experience both as an author and as a reviewer and has ideally spent a stretch on an Editorial Board, not necessarily of the same but at least a related journal. During such a learning period, numerous connections and acquaintances can be made which come in useful as potential reviewers. The scene is familiar to him and vice versa.

As in any other profession, different personalities can be encountered: from the insensitive but highly efficient bureaucrat to the jovial and generous grandfather figure. It is easy to guess who will have the higher rejection rate and is more likely to wiggle through the thorny underbrush of scientific publishing unharmed. It is helpful for reviewers to know a bit about the psyche of the Editor in question, the problem being that they normally never meet in person. Thus, they are often left with speculations drawn from the final decisions made and the style of correspondence received.

If a reviewer does not perform to the satisfaction of an Editor, he may be penalized by being dropped off the list. If that seems to have happened and you would like to continue reviewing, just ask what is going on. You may simply have been shoved into a remote recess of memory. Remember that Editors tend to be senior in many senses of the word and bear in mind that the reviewer pool can easily have more than a hundred members, even in a smaller journal. The manuscript submission systems offer the Editor search functions for reviewers by name, keywords, location, etc., but the run-of-the-mill daily assignments are often simply made by thinking "This could interest good old Archie. Let's send it to him." A conscientious Editor should, however, keep track of the assignments across the year, thus avoiding Archie ending up with 20 invitations and feeling slightly overwhelmed, and cousin Wilma getting none despite of her meticulous two-page elaboration on that tricky molecular biology paper with the wonky statistics 10 months ago.

A good Editor should be open to everybody related to the journal and try to understand the often diverging interests. This is where the "-in-Chief" comes in. Although time consuming, this central position and the various challenges make the job so appealing to the enthusiastic ones.

10.2 The Editorial Board

If reviewing is something you really like and if you get positive feedback from the Editor, you may strive to become a member of the Editorial Board. Commonly, its members are recruited from exceptional reviewers as well as from experts for special aspects (statistics, related disciplines), so here is a chance to be promoted. The board should meet physically at least once a year to discuss the development of the journal as well as the solutions for potential problems. It is also the forum to present new ideas to and meant to be a professional advisory panel for difficult decisions and strategic development.

Becoming a board member carries obligations such as receiving more invitations to review or being asked for an additional opinion in cases of controversy. Attending the meetings regularly is also expected. Depending on the structure of the journal, members may also be asked to subedit a special issue or supplement. This can be regarded as training for an editorial position and should therefore be taken seriously.

Again, it is the Editor's task to survey the Board on a regular basis for efficiency and diversity. Many journals limit the time-span for board members to ensure a turn-over.

10.3 Society Representatives

In journals which are the scientific publications of learned societies, it is normal for executives of that society to have a place on the board. As being, for instance, an outgoing president does not necessarily qualify that person to be a proficient and experienced reviewer or much-needed expert, the Editor may decide to host a special subsection of the board called "Society Representatives" or similar. With the journal being a showcase of the society, it is one of the responsibilities of these representatives to watch if published content openly contradicts official policies of the society. It must, on the other hand, be absolutely clear that the Editor-in-Chief has an independent function, meaning independent of the owner, the society, the authors, the reviewers, the own employer, etc. Conflicts of interest can arise and have led to dismissal or resignation of Editors.

😕 Bad Example

If, for instance, the Bavarian Society of Asphaltology has published a statement that it does not endorse the CARB-2 regimen for the treatment of grade III asphaltoma, and the

Editor of the *Bavarian Journal of Asphaltology* keeps accepting manuscripts proposing just that, this situation may become problematic.

Whereas the Editor must have freedom of opinion and may act following strict scientific selection criteria, the approach of the society that has its logo on the cover must also be respected. An open discussion between the Society Representatives and the Editorial Board should produce a solution acceptable for all.

10.4 Owner

It is very common for a journal to be "owned" by the publishing house. This means that the publisher has the rights on the title of the journal and that the Editor or a learned society cannot change publishers or even the design and setup at random.

😞 Bad Example

The Bavarian Society of Asphaltology, having realized that its contract with Bauer Publishers is about to end next year, has contacted Manalishi Scientific Journals for a competitive offer. Their conditions do look very appealing. Bauer informs them that they are free to change publishers, but that the title *Bavarian Journal of Asphaltology* is not for sale. This comes as a nasty surprise to the society, because it means that the new journal needs a different and unfamiliar name, will start from scratch, won't have a Journal Impact Factor for the next years, will therefore not be particularly attractive for authors, etc. Considering that they are happy to stay with Bauer.

Reviewers are usually not affected by these legal intricacies. They should, however, be aware of whom they are actually "working for" because it is the owner who is responsible for the manuscript submission system, etc.

10.5 Rewards

Being a reviewer can be a thankless task. As so often in science, it is taken for granted that the invited one feels an obligation to agree, may need it to boost the CV, wants to endear himself to the Editor/society, and should be grateful to be part of the chosen people anyway. What most journals do is to publish a lukewarm thank-you message once a year covering everybody who has been active the year before. Hit lists such as the "10 Best Reviewers in 2018" must be controversial, may cause considerable discontent among those not on it, and will always be a subjective selection, usually by the Editor. To avoid nerve-wrecking vanity discussions such awards tend not to be published, in turn diminishing their value.

Depending on the environment, journals may be in the position to offer CME credit points for every review performed, a popular incentive. An Editor-colleague in Scotland, obviously commanding an impressive budget, sends out a plate of smoked salmon at Christmas.

More recently, an initiative called Publons (https://publons.com) has gained considerable interest. Reviewers can register with a database, keep track of their reviews, and make themselves known to journals worldwide also subscribing to the system. Editors of affiliated journals can review their history and may choose to invite them for their own purposes. The system also helps to administer publications, citation metrics, and much more. The Publons Academy offers a training course in reviewing for registered members, the number of which seems to increase rapidly. Publons is certainly one of the most interesting developments in peer review in the last years.

Perhaps the most valuable reward you get for reviewing manuscripts is that you constantly learn by doing so. You learn about the content of the research reported but must keep in mind that all information is confidential until publication. You also keep learning about writing papers. Even if you are very experienced, you will still encounter a particularly original presentation or way of phrasing worth knowing (in good manuscripts) or, conversely, obvious blunders to avoid (in bad ones). In the end this will make you an even better author yourself.

11

Final Note

Reviewing a scientific paper is a bit like writing one. There are certain formalities to be followed, there are a lot of hidden traps to fall into, and the reward remains uncertain.

Just like workshops for authors, you can find numerous courses and instructions for reviewers by various publishers and journals, some of them comprehensive, some of them more like checklists. Several served as inspirations for the pages you just read. If there are issues not covered or if some advice given is considered controversial, please let me know (editorthcvs@thieme.com). Like science, the whole effort is a learning system.

This little booklet is supposed to help you in an entertaining way, and I hope you enjoyed reading it. If you will happily remember some of the examples the next time you sit down to review a manuscript, it will have served its purpose.

12

References

1. Heinemann MK. How NOT to Write a Medical Paper: A Practical Guide. 2nd ed. Delhi, Stuttgart, New York, Rio de Janeiro, Beijing: Thieme Publishers; 2018
2. Bravo G, Grimaldo F, Lopez-Inesta E, Mehmani B, Squazzoni F. The effect of publishing peer review reports on referee behavior in five scholarly journals. Nature Comm 2019;10:322–329
3. Leopold SS, Haddad FS, Sandell LJ, Swiontkowski M. Clinical orthopaedics and related research, The Bone & Joint Journal, the Journal of Orthopaedic Research, and The Journal of Bone and Joint Surgery will not accept clinical research manuscripts previously posted to preprint servers. J Bone Joint Surg Am 2019;101:1–4
4. Stahel PF, Moore EE. How to review a surgical paper: a guide for junior referees. BMC Med 2016;14:29
5. https://publicationethics.org/files/Ethical_Guidelines_For_Peer_Reviewers_2.pdf
6. https://www.salon.com/2018/10/01/how-a-failed-psoriasis-study-pushed-a-whole-field-forward_partner/

7. Regazzi JJ, Selenay A. Author-perceived quality characteristics of science, technology and medicine (STM) journals. ALPSP 2008

Index